I0486074

Midwifery Client File

Client Name:

EDD:

ACCOUNT LEDGER

Name: _____ Phone: _____

Address: _____

Initial service date: _____ EDD: _____

Agreements

Agreed Fee: _____ Non-Refundable Deposit: _____ Assistant Fee: _____

Services to include: _____

Payment Plan: _____

Miscellaneous

Assistant Fee and Date Paid: _____

Other Fee and Date Paid: _____

DATE	DESCRIPTION	CASH	CHECK #	AMOUNT	BALANCE DUE

Registration Form

_____ _____ _____
Name of Client (First/Middle/Last)   (Maiden)   Date of Birth

_____ _____
Father's Name (First/Middle/Last)   Father's Date of Birth

_____ _____
Client's Occupation   Father's Occupation

_____
Complete Address

_____
Mailing Address (if different)

(_____)_____ (_____)_____ (_____)_____
Home Phone   Cellular Phone   Other (specify):

_____
E-mail Address

_____ _____
Insurance Carrier   Policy Number and Date of Effectiveness

Are you the primary insured? _____ If not who is? _____ Relationship_____

_____
Insurance Address

(_____)_____
Insurance Phone

In case of an emergency, is there anyone you would want us to contact? Please list their contact information/phone numbers:

_____

_____

_____

_____

_____

Personal GYN History for _____

Menstrual History

How often do you menstruate? _____days
Is your flow ☐ scant ☐ moderate ☐ heavy ☐ regular ☐ irreg
If irregular, please explain
_____
_____
How old were you when you started menstruating?_____
Do you have cramps? YES NO ☐ mild ☐ moderate ☐ severe
When was your last menstrual period?_____
Was it normal?_____
Are you aware of the date you conceived?_____

Gynecological & Birth Control History

When was your last pap smear?_____
Have you ever had an abnormal pap smear? YES NO_____
_____
Have you ever had   infertility_____   vag inf_____
  abnormal bleeding_____   breast surgery_____
  cervical surgery_____   uterine surgery_____
  Any STDs_____
Do you feel that you might be at risk for any STDs? YES NO
_____
Most recent birth control used_____
Contraception used in the past; what, when, any problems?
_____
_____

Sexual History

Are you sexually active YES NO
Do you have painful intercourse? YES NO Bleeding? YES NO
How would you describe your sexual relationship?_____
_____
How do you feel your sexual relationship has changed since
you got pregnant?_____
_____
Have you had more than one partner? YES NO
Have you ever had non consensual sex? YES NO
If so, do you feel that experience will affect have an affect on
your labor/birth?_____

Was this a planned pregnancy? YES NO
What are your feelings about it?_____
Your spouse's/partner's feelings?_____

Anything else?

Anything else you would like me to know?

Client's Pregnancy History (list all pregnancies and outcomes)

DOB	Name	M/F	How many weeks	Weight	Hours Labor	c-sec/ vbac	Any issues or complications during pregnancy or birth?

Problems in Current Pregnancy

☐ 1st trimester nausea_____
☐ 2nd/3rd trimester nausea_____
☐ Varicose veins_____
☐ Bladder infections_____
☐ Kidney infections_____
☐ Spotting/Bleeding_____
☐ Premature labor_____
☐ Anemia_____

☐ Constipation_____
☐ Hemorrhoids_____
☐ Headaches_____
☐ Dizziness_____
☐ Swelling_____
☐ Gastritis_____
☐ Heartburn_____
☐ Any trauma_____

Exposures in Current Pregnancy

☐ Tobacco_____
☐ Alcohol_____
☐ Caffeine_____
☐ Marijuana_____
☐ Cocaine_____
☐ Street Drugs_____
☐ Other meds_____
☐ Non-pres.drugs_____

☐ Vitamins_____
☐ Fumes/sprays_____
☐ Enviro Toxins_____
☐ X-rays_____
☐ Measles/Viruses_____
☐ Vaccinations_____
☐ Cats_____
☐ Other_____

Social History

Do you enjoy your work? YES NO _____

Describe your stress level_____

_____

What do you do to relax or relieve stress?_____

Do you exercise? YES NO How often?_____ How long?_____

Tobacco Use ☐ None Packs/Day_____ How long?_____

Do you want to quit smoking? YES NO

Street Drug Use ☐ None Drug_____ How often?_____

Alcohol Use ☐ None # Drinks/Day/Week/Month_____

Have you ever been or are you now in an abusive relationship? YES NO

Has anyone now, or in the past :

Hit, kicked or pushed you? YES NO

 Verbally abused you? YES NO

Do you feel safe in your current relationship? YES NO

EMOTIONAL RISK ASSESSMENT

Are you a nervous person? YES NO

Do you often feel sad or depressed? YES NO

Do you feel a desire to hurt others? YES NO

Do you often feel angry or upset? YES NO

Do you feel a desire to hurt yourself? YES NO

Have you recently suffered a major loss/change? YES NO

Is there anything else you feel could be helpful to us in providing your care? _____

Client's Medical History

Allergies to any medications?_____ Reactions_____

Have you ever had a blood transfusion? YES NO   Any uterine surgeries? _____

List any other injuries, surgery, or hospitalization with dates_____

Check all that apply:

☐ Asthma_____
☐ Diabetes_____
☐ Drug addiction_____
☐ Heart disease_____

☐ Seizures_____
☐ Thrombophlebitis_____
☐ Chronic Hypertension_____
☐ Renal disease_____

☐ Auto immune disorders____
☐ Cancer_____
☐ TB_____
☐ Thyroid disorder_____

☐ Liver problems_____
☐ Blood disorders_____
☐ HIV / Hepatitis_____
☐ Syphilis_____

Risk Assessment

In this or one of your previous pregnancies have you had:

YES NO Severe hyperemesis requiring hospitalization

YES NO Preterm rupture of membranes (<36 wks)

YES NO Shoulder dystocia, resulting in trauma to the baby

YES NO Placenta abruption

YES NO Placenta previa

YES NO Gestational diabetes (controlled)

YES NO RH sensization

YES NO Medical disorders or endocrine, renal, cardiac or
        vascular systems

YES NO Postpartum hemorrhage (requiring bl transfusion)

YES NO Pelvic/genital tract abnormalities

YES NO Suspected cervical incompetence

YES NO Inverted uterus

YES NO Recurrent UTI's

YES NO Are you or the FOB related by blood?

YES NO   Are your or the FOB from any of these ethnic/racial
groups? Jewish Black/African Asian Mediterranean

Family's Medical History

Father: Alive and well? YES NO_____ Mother: Alive and well? YES NO_____ Siblings: Alive and well? YES NO_____

Check all that apply:

☐ Hypertension_____
☐ Kidney problems_____
☐ Diabetes_____

☐ Heart disease_____
☐ Blood disorders_____
☐ TB_____

☐ Allergies_____
☐ Twins_____
☐ Genetic anomalies_____

☐ Downs syndrome_____
☐ Cancer_____
☐ Other_____

Client Health Record Checklist

Name _____   EDD _____

INITIAL VISIT

_____ Draw Labs
_____ AFP ☐ Declined ☐ To do
_____ CF ☐ Declined ☐ To do
_____ Genetic Counseling, PRN
_____ Diet History
_____ Danger Signs
_____ Habits: smoking, ETOH, drugs
_____ Exercise; sexuality
_____ Discomforts
_____ Financial Agreement
_____ Consent Forms

16-20 WEEKS

_____ Schedule US, PRN
_____ Draw/Decline AFP

24-28 WEEKS

_____ Draw/Decline GT
_____ HCT
_____ AB screen PRN
_____ Rhogam PRN
_____ PTL Signs
_____ Childbirth Class
_____ Breastfeeding

30-32 WEEKS

_____ Labor Support
_____ Danger Signs: ROM, headache, visual disturbances, etc

34-36 WEEKS

_____ Obtain/Decline Group B Strep
_____ Supplies & preparation list

36 WEEKS

_____ Signs of Labor
_____ When and How to Call
_____ Pediatrician
_____ Supplies
_____ PP Support
_____ Breastfeeding
_____ Ready for Baby
_____ Back-up Plan/Map
_____ Newborn Screen Information

Continues to Meet Risk Criteria for Birth Home
(Weekly Evaluation)

36	37	38	39	40	41	42
☐	☐	☐	☐	☐	☐	☐

40-42 WEEKS

_____ Post-dates Routine
_____ NST
_____ Kick Count

RECORDS

Records Requested: _____
Records Received: _____

Lab Tests and Results

Client ID

Client Name

Date and Time	Tests Ordered	Results Received Date	Results

Lab Tests and Results

Client ID

Client Name

Date and Time	Tests Ordered	Results Received Date	Results

Ultrasound Exams and Reults

Client ID

Client Name

Date and Time	Tests Ordered	Results Received Date	Results

Client Name		Age		Meds		Allergies/Reaction	
		Height					
Date of Birth		Weight					
		LMP					
G P SAB TAB L		BP					
Reason for Visit		Hgb				Food:	
		Tobacco Y N					

Interval History

Physical Exam   Date   Initials

Gen Health	Physical		Height	Weight		BMI
	Emotional/Abuse/DV		Blood Pressure	Pulse		Temp

HEENT	Head ❑WNL	Lymph Glands ❑WNL	**Eyes**	Sclera ❑WNL
	Neck ❑WNL	Ears ❑WNL		Conjunctiva ❑WNL
	Thyroid ❑WNL	Nose/Mouth ❑WNL		Pupil Reaction ❑WNL

Chest

Breast Exam ❑Performed ❑Taught ❑Monthly BSE Advised ❑Discussed Mammograms ❑Nipples Checked
Comments:

Heart	Rate	Rhythm	Sounds	**Lungs**	Respiration Rate	Sounds

Abdomen & Back

Bowel Sounds	Spleen	Liver	Masses	Diastasis FB	Scars
Inguinal Nodes	Femoral Pulses	CVAT		Kidneys	Spine

Fundal Height CM	Placental Sounds (o)	Fetal Motion	FHT BPM	Fetal Position	Location of FHT

Extre-mities

Edema	Lesions	Reflexes	Clonus	Varicose Veins	Joint Range of Motion	Bruises

Skin

Tone	Lesions	Lumps	Color	Rash	Hair	Nails

Genitourinary

External	Internal
Scars ❑Y ❑N	Uterus ❑Anteflexed ❑Retroflexed
Prolapse ❑Y ❑N	❑ Normal Size, Shape, Contour
Discharge ❑Y ❑N	Cervix ❑WNL ❑ PAP Performed
Erythema ❑Y ❑N	Ovaries Palpable ❑Y ❑N ❑Possible Cyst
Sx of STDs/Infection ❑Y ❑N	Vagina ❑Cystocele ❑Rectocele ❑WNL
Anus/Rectum ❑WNL Lesions/Scars/Fissures/Hemorrhoids/Inflammation	
Comments	

Assessment

Plan

Midwife   **Assistants**

Prenatal Record

Mother _____

Partner _____

Children _____

Special Concerns & Considerations

_____

_____

_____

| G | P | T | P | Sa | Ea | L |

LMP _____

EDD: (N/W/US) _____

DOB _____

Blood Type _____

Allergies _____

Pre-pregnancy Weight _____

DATE	WEEKS	WEIGHT	BP/PULSE	FUNDUS	POSITION	FHT	MOVE MENT	URINE Pr/Gl/WBC		RETURN VISIT	INITIALS
									BA Bleeding Discharge Dizzy Edema Elimination Fatigue Gastric HA Mood N&V Sleep Vision Varicosities UC Urine		
									BA Bleeding Discharge Dizzy Edema Elimination Fatigue Gastric HA Mood N&V Sleep Vision Varicosities UC Urine		
									BA Bleeding Discharge Dizzy Edema Elimination Fatigue Gastric HA Mood N&V Sleep Vision Varicosities UC Urine		
									BA Bleeding Discharge Dizzy Edema Elimination Fatigue Gastric HA Mood N&V Sleep Vision Varicosities UC Urine		
									BA Bleeding Discharge Dizzy Edema Elimination Fatigue Gastric HA Mood N&V Sleep Vision Varicosities UC Urine		
									BA Bleeding Discharge Dizzy Edema Elimination Fatigue Gastric HA Mood N&V Sleep Vision Varicosities UC Urine		
									BA Bleeding Discharge Dizzy Edema Elimination Fatigue Gastric HA Mood N&V Sleep Vision Varicosities UC Urine		
									BA Bleeding Discharge Dizzy Edema Elimination Fatigue Gastric HA Mood N&V Sleep Vision Varicosities UC Urine		
									BA Bleeding Discharge Dizzy Edema Elimination Fatigue Gastric HA Mood N&V Sleep Vision Varicosities UC Urine		
									BA Bleeding Discharge Dizzy Edema Elimination Fatigue Gastric HA Mood N&V Sleep Vision Varicosities UC Urine		
									BA Bleeding Discharge Dizzy Edema Elimination Fatigue Gastric HA Mood N&V Sleep Vision Varicosities UC Urine		
									BA Bleeding Discharge Dizzy Edema Elimination Fatigue Gastric HA Mood N&V Sleep Vision Varicosities UC Urine		
									BA Bleeding Discharge Dizzy Edema Elimination Fatigue Gastric HA Mood N&V Sleep Vision Varicosities UC Urine		

Prenatal Follow Up Sheet for _____

G_____ P_____ A_____ L_____ EDD_____ Revised_____

Date	Issues Discussed	Midwife	Student

Prenatal Follow Up Sheet for _____

G_____ P_____ A_____ L_____ EDD_____ Revised_____

Date	Issues Discussed	Midwife	Student

Prenatal Follow Up Sheet for _____

G_____ P_____ A_____ L_____ EDD_____ Revised_____

Date	Issues Discussed	Midwife	Student

Labour Initial Intake

Client Name:_____**Phone#**:_____

Significant Issues:_____

Age:_____ **Gest. Wks**:_____ G/P:_____ EDD:_____ **Blood Type**:_____

SROM:_____ **Time**:_____ **Colour**:_____ **Odour**:_____ Show:_____

Time CTX Began:_____ Spacing:_____ Lasting:_____Coping:_____

Eating:_____ Drinking:_____ Time Last Eaten: _____Voiding:_____ BM:_____

TEMP	PULSE	BP	FHT	FUNDUS	POSITION	OTHER
					Movement	

Client's Concerns:_____
_____
_____

Notes

Midwife Staying?:_____ Transport to Hosp.?:_____
Early Labour Handout Given:_____ Has Labour/Birth Supplies:_____
Support People:_____

Prenatal Issues		
BP Range:	**BP Limits:**	**Any s/s PIH?**
Consults:	Completed:	Outstanding:
Hemo:	Varicosities:	**Labs WNL:**
FHR Range:	Fetal Probs:	Other:
Emotional:	Nutr./Vits.:	Hx of SA/Mol:
# Appts:	Complied Recos:	All Waivers Signed:

Client Name					Partner				Midwife		
Allergies						Blood Type	GBS Status + - ?		Assistant(s)		
G	**P**	SAB	TAB	L	VBAC Y N		LMP			EDD	

Onset of Labor	Date/Time	Contractions	Membranes	Show	Fetal Movement	Time MW Called	Comments

Assessment at Arrival	Date/Time	Contractions		Membranes	Show	Fetal Movement	Comments
	B/P	Pulse	Temp	Internal Exam	Activity/Rest/Food/Drink		

Time	B/P	Pulse	Temp	FHT **Rate** **Variability** **Location**	IN	Out	Contractions		Internal Exam **Dilation** **Station** **Effacement** **Position**	Comments	Initials
							Frequency (Minutes)	Duration (Seconds)			

Client Name					Date				Midwife/Students		

Time	B/P	Pulse	Temp	FHT	IN	Out	Contractions		Internal Exam	Comments	Initials
				Rate Variability Location			Frequency (Minutes)	Duration (Seconds)	Dilation Station Effacement Position		

| Client Name | | | | | Date | | | | Midwife/Students | | |

Time	B/P	Pulse	Temp	FHT	IN	Out	Contractions		Internal Exam	Comments	Initials
				Rate Variability Location			Frequency (Minutes)	Duration (Seconds)	Dilation Station Effacement Position		

Labor Notes for _____

Baby's Name_____ Date of Birth_____

Date	Issues Discussed	Midwife	Student

Labor Notes for _____

Baby's Name_____ Date of Birth_____

Date	Issues Discussed	Midwife	Student

Labor Notes for _____

Baby's Name_____ Date of Birth_____

Date	Issues Discussed	Midwife	Student

Immediate Postpartum Record

Date:_____ Time of birth:_____ am/pm

Client's Status (name)_____

Time	Vitals			Uterus PBL_____cups/cc		In/Out	Comments	Init
Hour am/pm	Pulse	Temp	B/P	Status	Blood loss	Intake, etc	Notes	Initials

Baby's Status (name)_____

Time	Vitals			In/Out		Comments	Init
Hour am/pm	Pulse	Resp	Temp	Intake	Output	Notes	Initials

Total time of postpartum care_____ Total estimated blood loss_____

Discharged from Midwife's care on_____ at _____am/pm MW_____

Newborn Exam

Baby's Name			Mother's Name			
Date		**Time**	**APGAR**	**1 Minute**	**5 Minutes**	**Sign**
Gender	**Weight**	**Length**	Heart Rate			0 = Absent 1 = Below 100 2 = Above 100
OFC	**Chest**	**EGA**	Respiratory Effort			0 = Absent 1 = Slow, Irregular 2 = Good crying
Respirations	**Heart Rate**	**Temp**	Muscle Tone			0 = Flaccid 1 = Some flexion of extremities 2 = Active motion
Birth Time	**Midwife**		Color			0 = Pale blue 1 = Body pink, extremities blue 2 = Completely pink
General Appearance (activity, tone, cry)			Reflex Irritability			0 = None 1 = Grimace 2 = Vigorous Cry
			Total Score			

Skin (polycythemia, jaundice desquamation, lanugo, birth marks)

Head. Neck (molding, caput, bruising, cephalhematoma, fontanelles)

Eyes (red spots, jaundice, pupils, tracking)	Erythromycin Ointment
ENT (ear placement, reactivity to sound, lips, palate, frenulum)	Hips (clicks, creases)
Thorax (retractions) Present? Y / N	Abdomen (cord, masses)
Heart	Femoral Pulses
Genitals (testes descended, edema, labia, clitoris)	Spine/Anus (sinuses, anus patent)
Lungs	Extremities (fingers, toes, clavicles)

Reflexes

Babinski	Present?	Y / N	Sucking	Present?	Y / N	Comments
Palmar	Present?	Y / N	Swallowing	Present?	Y / N	
Plantar	Present?	Y / N	Step	Present?	Y / N	
Moro	Present?	Y / N	Tonic Neck	Present?	Y / N	

Gestational Age Assessment (in weeks)	**Preterm**				**Term**				**Post-term**	
	34	35	36	37	38	39	40	41	42	43+
Vernix	Covers body, thick layer				Back, scalp, in creases		Scant in creases		No vernix	
Breast Tissue and Areola	Areola raised		1-2 mm nodule		3-5 mm	5-6 mm	7-10 mm			
Ear Form	Beginning incurving superior		Incurving upper 2/3 pinnae		Well-defined incurving to lobe					
Ear Cartilage	Scant, ret. slowly from folding		Thin, springs back from folding			Pinnae firm, remains erect from head				
Sole Creases	1-2 ant.	2-3 ant.	Anterior 2/3 sole		Involving heel				Entire sole	
Skin (thickness and appearance)	Smooth, no edema			Thicker, no desquamation, few vessels			Some desquamation		Thick, desq entire body	
Nail plates	Nails to fingertips								Well past tips	
Hair	Fine/wooly, bunches out from head				Silky single strands, lays flat				Receding	
Lanugo	None on face, present on body				Present on shoulders				No lanugo	
Labia & Clitoris	Prominent clitoris, labia small, widely separated			Labia majora larger, nearly cover clitoris			Labia minora and clitoris covered			
Testes	Palpable in inguinal canal			In upper scrotum			In lower scrotum			
Scrotum	Few rugae			Rugae anterior portion			Rugae cover		Pendulous	
Skull firmness	Soft to 1" from ant fontanelle		Spongy at edges of fontanelle, center firm		Bones hard, sutures easily displaced				Hard, can't displace	

Examiner's Signature

Placenta Examination Form

Name of Mother_____ EDD: _____

Name of Infant _____

Date of birth _____ Time of birth: _____

Significant health history _____

_____

Brief summary of the birth _____

Length of 3rd stage_____

Method of placental birth:

      Spontaneous _____ Assisted _____ Extracted _____

If extracted, state reasons, method and outcome

_____

_____

Were oxytocic's, either herbal or pharmacological used for postpartum bleeding or to release the placenta?

Yes _____ No _____ If yes, what and why

_____

_____

    Dose_____ Frequency _____

    Results: _____

Total blood loss _____
Before birth of placenta _____
After birth of placenta _____

Retroplacental clots _____ Size _____ Number _____ Placement _____
Approximate age of clots _____ Size and weight _____

Notes:

_____

_____

_____

Placenta Weight _____
Circumference _____
Thickness _____
Color _____

Any signs or symptoms of infection _____ Odor _____ Pallor _____ Other
_____

Maternal (Duncan) side:
Color _____
Consistency: Normal _____ Soft _____ Firm _____
If not complete describe: _____
Overall impression: Infarcts, calcification, abnormalities of the vascular bed, nodes
etc.
_____
_____
_____

Baby's side (Shultz): Overall impression
_____
_____
_____

 Note obvious variations or abnormalities of shape
_____
_____

Extraplacental membranes:
Are the membranes complete: Yes ___ No ___
Presence of Amnion _____
Presence of Chorion _____
Evidence of amniotic web syndrome _____
Point of rupture: Evidence of low lying placental implantation: Yes ____ No ____
Circummarginate _____
Circumvallate _____

Umbilical cord: Site of insertion:
Central _____
Eccentric _____
Battledore _____
      If it is a battledore insertion, where is the point of rupture _____
Velamentous _____
Furcate insertion _____
Evidence of Vasa Previa _____

Cord length _____
True knot(s) _____
False knot(s) _____
Webbing _____
Presence of Warton's jelly _____
Thrombosis _____
Single artery _____ If yes, which artery is missing: right _____ left _____
Chirality of cord: right spiral ___ left spiral ___ none _____ excessive _____
Edema of the cord: Yes ___ No ___
Nuchal cord _____

Sketch a diagram of anything of note:

Overall health and well-being of this newborn

_____
_____
_____
_____

Any evidence of problems with this newborn related to anomalies within this placenta: Yes ___ No ___
If yes explain:

_____
_____
_____
_____

Photographs taken for documentation _____

Referral or consultation: Yes _____ No _____
If yes, with whom _____

_____   _____
Signature of attending midwife   Date

_____   _____
Signature of Consultant – if consult done   Date

Please note: Obvious abnormalities of the placenta may warrant further examination by a pathologist. If you feel that there may be a need for this, do not freeze the placenta. Dry it well, place it in a zip lock bag removing all of the air possible and then place it into an air tight plastic container. Tape it closed with red tape. This is a safe way to transport "Hazardous Biological Waste" if you need to take it for examination to a hospital. Freezing the placenta changes the tissues altering the pathologist's ability to do accurate microscopic examinations.

Client's Name_____ Date Birth_____

	36-48 hours	5 days	2 weeks	4-6 weeks
Time/ Date				
T | P | BP				
Feedings milk in nipples sore engorged redness	Breast _____ Formula_____	Breast _____ Formula_____	Breast _____ Formula_____	Breast _____ Formula_____
Involution after pains				
Locia abn odor	#_____ of kotex day Rubra Serosa Alba	#_____ of kotex day Rubra Serosa Alba	#_____ of kotex day Rubra Serosa Alba	#_____ of kotex day Rubra Serosa Alba
Perineum				
Elimination void / BM hemorrhoids discomfort				
Hygiene				
Condition		Hemo_____	Hemo_____	
Midwife				

Baby's Name_____ Wt at birth ___lbs ___oz ____grams

General Condition				
Weight				
Color/Skin				
Umbilicus				
Voiding/BM				
Midwife				
PKU	Date done_____ Days postpartum_____ With whom_____ Results_____			

Postpartum Follow Up Sheet for _____

Baby's Name_____ Date of Birth_____

Date	Issues Discussed	Midwife	Student

Postpartum Follow Up Sheet for _____

Baby's Name_____ Date of Birth_____

Date	Issues Discussed	Midwife	Student

Postpartum Follow Up Sheet for _____

Baby's Name_____ Date of Birth_____

Date	Issues Discussed	Midwife	Student

STATEMENT OF BIRTH

Date of Birth: _____/_____/_____ Time of Birth: _____

Address of Birth: _____

Child's Name: _____ Gender: _____

Mother's Name: _____ Age: _____

Attendant's Name and Title: _____

WITNESSES OTHER THAN ATTENDANT: (If any)

1) Name:_____

    Address: _____

    Relationship to Mother: _____

2) Name:_____

    Address: _____

    Relationship to Mother: _____

I, _____ do hereby swear that all information given in this document is true and accurate to the best of my knowledge.

Date: _____

Attendant Signature: _____

Mother Signature: _____

Witness 1 – Signature: _____

Witness 2 – Signature: _____

Attendant Contact Info:

Name: _____ Phone: _____ Fax: _____

Address:

Summary of Labor, Birth, Immediate Postpartum & Newborn

Client _____

G___ **P**___SAB___TAB___L___ VBAC ___ EDD_____ Wks_____ GBS_____ Total Weight Gain:_____

First Stage Summary

Onset latent labor ____/____/____ ____am/pm ____hrs ____min

Onset active labor ____/____/____ ____am/pm ____hrs ____min

Comments:

ROM at ____/____/____ ____am/pm
until delivery ____hrs ____min
Confirmed by □ visual □ nitrazine □ fetal hair □ fern □ referral
Labor Aids
□ ambulant □ positional □ nipple stim □ water □ castor oil
□ enema □ homeopathics □ herbs □ other _____
Membranes □ SROM □ AROM why?_____
With– □ no ctx □ latent □ active □ 2nd stage □ in caul
Amount-- □ fetal hair □ fern □ referral
Condition– □ clear □ lt mec □ mod mec □ thick mec □ term mec

Second Stage Summary

Onset 2nd stage ____/____/____ ____am/pm ____hrs ____min

Birth of Baby ____/____/____ **Time of Birth** _____am/pm

Resuscitation/Suctioning □ None □ YES
□ DeLee   □ Bulb Syringe □ PPV ____ # of minutes

Comments:

Positions √ Pushed ■Delivered
□ squat □ stand □ H&K □ McRoberts □ knee/chest
□ lithotomy □ Simms □ on toilet □ waterbirth □ other_____
Presentation □ OA □ OP □ Other _____
Nuchal Arm □ none x_____ **Nuchal Cord** □ none x_____

Perineum □ TEAR □ EPIS □ intact □ <1 □ 1 □ 2 □ 3 □ 4
Labial Tear □ intact □ skids □ needed sutures
Repair □ YES □ NO
by_____

Third Stage Summary

Placenta Delivered ____/____/____ ____am/pm ____hrs ____min
Was Delivered □ spontaneously □ assisted □ manual removal
Placenta Birthed in □ Shultz □ Duncan
Placenta/Membranes □ complete □ incom □ unsure □ cord 3 vessel
Cond □ stained □ marginal □ velamentous □ TRUE/FALSE knots
□ calcifications □ small □ average □ large
Comments:

Herbs_____
                    @_____am/pm @_____am/pm

Estimated PBL _____cups/cc □ scant □ moderate □ heavy
                    (0-250cc/1c) (250-1000 cc/1-4 c) (>1000cc/4c)

Newborn Examination   ♀   ♂

Date of Examination_____ **Time** _____am/pm

Baby's Name _____

Weight ____lbs ____oz ____gm
Length____ **Chest**____ **OFC**____
GA by dates____ **EGA by exam**____wks

Eye Care (Erythromycin) □ refused □ administered time____am/pm
Vit K □ refused □ advised □ admin □ IM □ PO BY_____
Cord Blood □ blood type/rh □ RPR □ HIV □ Hep B □ other _____

Comments_____
Examination by_____ Apgars 1min____5min____

Reflexes □ moro □ plantar □ palmar □ Babinski □ suck
□ root/suck □ blink □ stepping

Physical Exam √ if WNL

□ gen appearance _____	□ nipples_____
□ skin/color_____	□ abdomen_____
□ fontanels_____	□ cord_____
□ head_____	□ spine_____
□ ears_____	□ anus_____
□ eyes_____	□ genitalia_____
□ nose_____	□ extremities_____
□ throat_____	□ hips_____
□ mouth_____	□ birth marks_____
□ clavicle_____	□ mongolian spot_____
□ heart_____	□ stork bite_____
□ lungs_____	

Client Discharged / Midwife Left

Date_____ **Time** _____am/pm ____hrs ____min pp

Total PPBL _____cups/cc **Midwife**_____
Comments:

Present @ Birth

Midwife_____

Asst_____

Others_____

Transport Summary

Client

Name_____ Age____ G___ P___ A___ L___ Phone (____)_____
Address_____ City _____ State_____ Zip_____
Emergency Contact _____ Phone (____)_____ Relation_____
LMP_____ EDD_____ Dates changed_____ by_____
Prenatal care began _____ @ _____wks Number of visits with MW___ other___
Blood type____ HBG____ Antibody screen____ RPR/VDRL____ Rubella____ Pap_____
GBS_____ GC/CT_____ HIV____ Heb B____ Glucose_____

Labor

Latent labor began Date_____ Time_____ am/pm FHR _____
Active labor began Date_____ Time_____ am/pm FHR _____
Rupture of membranes Date_____ Time_____ am/pm Color _____ INTACT
Assessment prior to transport: Temp_____ Pulse_____ Resps_____ B/P_____ Laceration_____
_____cm _____eff _____station Position of baby_____ Urine Prot____ Gluc____ Ket____ Nit____
Placenta time_____ am/pm Complete YES NO EBL _____cups/cc
Reason for transport_____
_____

Newborn

Date of Birth_____ Time_____am/pm
Weight _____lbs _____oz _____grams
Meconium_____ Eye care_____ Vit K_____
Bulb_____Delee_____ Bag & mask_____ CPR_____
Reason for transport_____
_____
_____

Apgars of Baby

	1 min	5 min	10 min
Heart	0 1 2	0 1 2	0 1 2
Resps	0 1 2	0 1 2	0 1 2
Reflex	0 1 2	0 1 2	0 1 2
Tone	0 1 2	0 1 2	0 1 2
Color	0 1 2	0 1 2	0 1 2

Transport

_____Hospital contacted on_____ at _____am/pm DR_____
by EMS – Date called _____ at _____ am/pm Arrived @_____ departed @_____
by Private vehicle- departed on _____ at _____ am/pm Arrived @_____

Midwife's Name:_____ Signature_____

www.ingramcontent.com/pod-product-compliance
Lightning Source LLC
Chambersburg PA
CBHW080645180526
45168CB00008B/3312